THE WELLNESS EFFECT

Hidden Implications
of a Healthy Lifestyle

THE
WELLNESS
EFFECT

Hidden Implications
of a Healthy Lifestyle

Gene Clerkin, DC

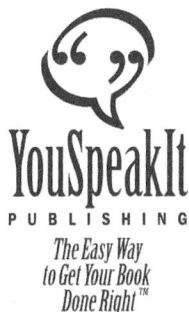

YouSpeakIt
PUBLISHING
*The Easy Way
to Get Your Book
Done Right*™

www.YouSpeakItPublishing.com

For my wife, Castine, for her endless love, support, and encouragement, and to my boys, Kaeran and Seamus, for keeping me young and helping me to see the wonders of life.

Contents

Acknowledgments   9

Introduction   13

CHAPTER ONE

Our Health—

  In Critical Condition   17

    Something's Wrong   17

    It's A Question Of Philosophy   25

    Symptomism   31

CHAPTER TWO

Why Is Health Declining?   39

  Stress   39

  Poor Choice   46

  Our Environment   54

  Frankenfoods   58

CHAPTER THREE

Health Impact   61

  Ouch, That Hurts!   61

  How Do You Feel About That?   66

  Breaking The Bank   72

CHAPTER FOUR

Steps To Regaining Health   77

  Awareness   77

Desire   84

The Road Map   89

CHAPTER FIVE

The Ripple Effect   95

  Personal Benefits Of Health

    And Wellness   95

  Beyond The Physical   100

  The Ripple Effect   105

Conclusion   111

Next Steps   115

About The Author   117

Acknowledgments

I'd first like to acknowledge my parents, Hugh and Melba Clerkin. My father came to this country as an Irish immigrant at the age of sixteen. As a do-it-yourselfer, he taught me the value of hard work and persistence. My mom showed me by example from her own life how to move through life's adversity and come out the other side.

Dr. Reggie Gold and Dr. Joe Strauss. Each heavily influenced my professional direction with their teachings on chiropractic philosophy and vitalistic thinking. Their teachings became the foundation and standard upon which everything else I learned was built. Both were dedicated to passing on their knowledge and mentoring countless doctors of chiropractic.

Dr. Donald Epstein, who has been on the forefront of developing technologies for human potential for over thirty years. I remember the first time I attended one of his seminars. He spoke about the wisdom of the body and symptoms as an intelligent response rather than a nuisance to be quelled. Epstein is never satisfied with the status quo and has encouraged thousands of doctors to move to higher levels of personal and professional growth, integrity, and purpose. He continues to be a pioneer in the development of human potential technologies.

If it weren't for Dr. Freddie Ulan and the systems he developed, my health would have continued to spiral downward. Dr. Ulan battled his own major health challenges and helped thousands of patients regain their own health as well. He then felt compelled to share his detail-oriented and systematic approach with thousands of doctors across the country. In addition to getting my own health back, I have been able to help so many patients of my own with his systems.

Dr. Charlie Webb has helped, and continues to help me reach so many more people than I ever could before. Dr. Webb is a master communicator and focuses on teaching doctors how to educate their patients to become self-empowered and gain their health independence. His purpose is to mentor as many doctors as he can, so they can reach and help as many patients as possible to positively impact the health of this country.

Thousands of clients and patients have placed their trust in me to help guide them on their healing journey. Because of them, I've had the opportunity to contribute my knowledge, experience, and clinical skills and center my life around helping others. There is no better feeling than being able to help someone regain their health and improve their quality of life.

While most patients come to their practitioners seeking knowledge and guidance, they also end up being the teachers. Much like relationships, professional practice is a vehicle for personal development. I thank you all for the past twenty-four years of growth and development.

Introduction

There are numerous books available on what to do to get well. A simple search on the internet yields countless websites teeming with information—energy work, nutrition, chiropractic, acupuncture, and endless others. Although the methods vary, most yield some degree of results.

Why then is health in our country in such a poor state?

It's great to have options for restoring and maintaining our health. But without having a game plan and acting to utilize these options in the appropriate fashion, we're destined to continue down the path of declining health.

In this book, we will explore:

- What's wrong, and what can you do about it?
- Why did you lose your health?
- Why is it worth investing your time, effort, and money to get your health back?

In the past twenty-four years, I have been working with clients who have varying degrees of health issues. Regardless of the complexity of the case, the formula for regaining health is quite similar. One major key is our lifestyle habits.

By making the necessary changes in health and lifestyle, you can dramatically improve your health. In addition to improving lifestyle, there is certainly a clinical piece to improving health. It's possible there is an underlying toxicity like mercury, or a hidden pathogen like an undetected parasite. But the clinical piece is secondary to making fundamental lifestyle changes.

Unfortunately, too many people simply don't make the changes that are necessary to restore and maintain their health. Sometimes, they don't know what to do, and if they do know, it far from guarantees that they will really do anything at all.

From my observations, many people either don't believe their lifestyle choices will make a difference, or they can't comprehend what it would look or feel like if they did. They don't necessarily consider or understand the impact that their state of health has on their own quality of life or how it affects others.

I wrote this book to inspire you to pursue a greater level of health and wellness. I want you to know that it is possible and will make a difference — not only for you, but also for the people you love and who love you. Finally, I'd like to share the powerful realization that the impact of our collective health choices will reshape and determine the landscape of our culture.

If you are reading this book and have been suffering with weight challenges, lack of energy, sleep issues, pain, or any other chronic health problems — *know that a slow deterioration of health and quality of life does not need to be your destiny.* If the only solution you've known is suppression of your symptoms with medications, know that there is an alternative. No matter where you are regarding your health, even if you think it's too late, you can always improve. I hope this book will inspire you to take the next step toward better health and a better quality of life.

CHAPTER ONE

Our Health—
In Critical Condition

SOMETHING'S WRONG

I can't imagine there is anyone out there who hasn't heard: *To be healthy, you must eat well and exercise.* Despite the simplicity and almost universal awareness of this advice, it hasn't translated to a healthy population.

A Sad State

When I was a kid, I remember seeing a commercial. In it, a Native American pulls his canoe up to a trash-riddled beach. As he walks around in disbelief, a bag of garbage is thrown at his feet from a passing car. The commercial ends with a tear running down his cheek. Obviously, he is distraught over what modern culture has done to his pristine environment. As I observe our modern society, it seems that the same heartless mentality that troubled the Native American has shaped almost every aspect of our culture.

It seems as if we don't care that our behaviors are destroying our environment and subsequently, our own health. We're just not aware of what we're doing. Regardless, the resulting outcomes of this cultural unconsciousness are plentiful and plain to see.

We're poisoning our environment and ourselves. Every year, tons of toxins are dumped into the environment. As the environment becomes more toxic, so do all its life forms — and that includes us. This is resulting in the extinction of many of our planet's species and a rapid decline in our health.

Here are some statistics from the CDC:

- Half the adults have a chronic disease.

- A quarter of adults have multiple chronic health conditions.
- Thirty percent of the children have a chronic health condition.

Chronic illnesses like heart disease, diabetes, cancer, and their myriad of physical symptoms are on the rise. This includes digestive disorders, such as acid reflux and bloating, and auto-immune disorders like Crohn's, rheumatoid arthritis, and eczema. But it's more than just the increase in pain or discomfort, or a decrease in energy at stake. Our mental and emotional health is declining as well.

Many Americans are suffering from mental disorders including depression, anxiety, memory loss, autism, and dementia. Mass shootings and the general state of violence in our society represent the decline of our collective mental health. The United States consistently ranks worst among industrialized nations in overall health, yet we spend more money than any country in the world. We are 5 percent of the world's population, yet we consume 50 percent of the world's medications.

We are putting all our resources into the traditional medical system with the expectation that it will protect our health, yet seven out of ten people in this country will wind up in a nursing home.

Does anyone really want to end up that way?

If we don't want to continue down this destructive path, we've got to take a close look at how we got here and use that to create a new roadmap.

The Healthcare System

The American healthcare system is a reactive system designed to manage or suppress symptoms without any real solutions for addressing the underlying problems. Sometimes, we hear the medical community talk about prevention, but it would be more accurate to call it early detection. If we are detecting something early, we didn't prevent it.

It's important to note that the standards in our traditional medical system are dictated by pharmaceutical and insurance companies. Once physicians detect disease, they must follow these standards of care or risk losing their license. Medical standards of care consist mostly of medications or surgery, even though these methods can never resolve the chronic health conditions that most Americans suffer with.

Why do most Americans continue to patronize a system that is obviously failing?

Part of the answer lies in health insurance.

But wait, isn't health insurance a good thing?

Sure, it's good to have insurance, but health insurance is unlike any other type of insurance. Most insurances are designed to be used for a crisis or emergency. For example, auto insurance is for when you have a car accident. You don't want to use it if you don't need to. Fire insurance is designed to protect your house in the event of a fire. Ideally, you never have to use it. The same would hold true for life insurance. You certainly wouldn't want to need to use that.

Health insurance is like buying a membership of benefits you can use. However, the only benefits available are pharmaceutical drugs and surgery. That tends to pigeon-hole people into one dimensional thinking when it comes to their health. Often, people develop a mindset that they can't pursue something different that might be beneficial because their insurance won't pay.

Most people think if they have health insurance their health will be protected. And, if everyone had health insurance, the overall health of the country would improve. While I'm not suggesting that one should not have health insurance for emergencies, it does little to help with the effects of chronic disease.

When I opened my private practice in 1994, I wanted to help as many people as I could. I began by placing a donation box on the wall, so people could pay whatever they could afford. What I found was health improvements were generally congruent with how much money people paid. If they paid very little or no money, their results were not as good.

If they valued their care and paid more, they tended to get better results. I've seen similar results with people who used their insurance. People who used insurance generally didn't achieve the same results as those who had to exchange their own hard-earned money for care. When people were personally investing in their care, results greatly improved.

A Social Directive

You must wonder why we think the way we do; but remember that most people in this country grew up watching TV.

I can recall — and most people do — slogans like: *Milk, it does the body good, Trix are for kids, and I'm cuckoo for Cocoa Puffs!* I can even recite the ingredients to a Big Mac: *two all-beef patties, special sauce, lettuce, cheese, pickles, onions on a sesame seed bun.*

Advertisements shape the way we think, the products we buy, the foods we eat, and ultimately what we do when we get sick. Pharmaceutical companies spend billions in advertising to convince people that medications are a normal way of life. And it works.

In an hour-long television show, you will see drug commercials repeated numerous times. Even though pharmaceutical companies must list all the side effects, they do it in a monotone voice, while simultaneously showing images of someone living a healthy, joyful life. People are suffering, so they make an emotional connection with the idea that life will be great when taking the medication. I think we all know it's not true.

These days, in addition to television, we also must contend with social media. You may have noticed that when you Google something, related advertisements begin to show up on your Facebook page. All our behaviors and interests are tracked to profile and ultimately direct our behaviors. We are profiled—and essentially brainwashed and directed—to continue to patronize a system that is clearly broken.

IT'S A QUESTION OF PHILOSOPHY

If we want to understand what is happening in our society, we must go to the root of how people think.

Let's Be Reasonable

There are two methods of reasoning: inductive and deductive.

- **Inductive reasoning** is based on gathering information and data, considering it, and reaching a conclusion.

- **Deductive reasoning** is based on the logical thought progression from a major premise or accepted idea, to concepts, and drawing a conclusion.

If the major premise is faulty, you can expect the ideas stemming from deductive reasoning will be false. Likewise, faulty bits or missing pieces of information render inductive reasoning ineffective. For example, there was a time when the accepted truth was that the world was flat. Of course, we now know the inductive conclusion based on the information available at the time was false.

It is worth noting that our healthcare system leans heavily toward inductive reasoning. *Physician's Desk Reference*, which is published by the pharmaceutical companies, lists all the information known about the medications they distribute, including the uses and side effects. It is interesting to note that the mode of action for almost all the medications listed is unknown. In other words: *they don't know how they work.*

Why not?

Because, as much information as we have learned about the human body, we still don't know much at all. If we did, our healthcare system might not be in such shambles.

Now what?

If we can't rely on compiled information or conflicting research studies, how are we supposed to make a healthy decision for ourselves or our children?

Using a combination of inductive and deductive reasoning, we must make conscious decisions based on what makes sense, not on what someone told us. Information is a good thing, but it must be used with wisdom and common sense.

A Vital Philosophy

Holistic and natural health practitioners tend to lean toward a vitalistic philosophy. In contrast, orthodox – or, the current medical system – leans toward a more mechanistic philosophy. More simply put, mechanists believe the body functions purely as a biochemical machine, whereas vitalists believe there is a life force animating the biochemical machine.

I recall being back in chiropractic school and working on cadavers. While staring in amazement at the masterpiece that is the human body, I remember clearly saying to myself, *Wow, there is no way this happened by mistake.* I believe this is one of the most defining moments of my belief system personally, spiritually, and professionally.

D.D. Palmer, who founded Chiropractic in 1895, based his philosophy on a major premise: "A universal intelligence is in all matter and continually gives to it all its properties and actions, thus maintaining it in existence."

In other words, without intelligence, matter could not exist. It may seem a little strange, but theists might unknowingly agree and call that universal intelligence God.

I have always liked the analogy that Dr. Reggie Gold shared to illustrate this principle: "If we found a watch on the side of the road, we could choose to believe that the elements and the structure of the watch came together randomly to create the intricate timepiece. While I suppose anything may be possible, I doubt most people would dispute that the watch was in fact designed and assembled by the watchmaker."

Why then, would we think the universe in its grandeur, or the human body for that matter, could be anything but designed intelligently?

Either the universe operates randomly or with intelligence as Palmer's premise supports. If you do support that premise, then it must logically apply to all levels of the web of life. Your decisions about how to interpret the body's symptoms and what actions to take are completely influenced by whether you trust what is happening.

In other words, when we exhibit symptoms, we must ask: *Should I trust that my body knows what it's doing?*

One of the greatest things about having a major philosophical premise to work from is that it can be applied to all situations, including how to eat, things to do for yourself, your relationship to the environment, and everything else.

People who are experiencing wellness tend to trust in the process of life. To me, the principle is a spiritual one that really applies to all aspects of life.

The question is: Do we trust the process, or are our life's labors met with fear and struggle?

There's No Cure for Healing

Even though we call it a healthcare system, our healthcare system is geared toward curing, not healing. Curing professionals, whether orthodox, medical, or even natural or alternative practitioners, concentrate on symptoms and normal tests. The focus is on curing the symptoms or moving lab test results. They seek to return the person to the state of health they were in before the symptoms occurred. But that was also the state of health that led to the symptomatic state in the first place.

Healing professions believe the body works intelligently and automatically moves toward health and healing if there isn't anything getting in the way. In the healing realm, practitioners generally want to help raise a person's health beyond what they were previously experiencing.

It's important to understand that curing is not a bad thing; sometimes it is necessary in a crisis to save a life. Curing can also be a stepping stone toward healing. The problem, through our cultural conditioning, is that we have come to believe that curing is healing. *That is why we call our system a healthcare system when it is really a disease detection and management system.*

SYMPTOMISM

Symptomism is a word I resurrected to describe our cultural conditioning and how we view our symptoms, not only in our body but also in life in general and how we address them.

What's the Meaning of This?

As previously mentioned, our traditional healthcare system focuses on the suppression of symptoms without full consideration of their purpose. This thought process has in-turn infiltrated our culture.

What is the first thing that comes to mind if we have a fever?

We've got to bring the fever down — but, why?

A fever can be a little uncomfortable, but it's exactly what the body needs when fighting an infection.

What about a skin rash?

Most people use a topical steroid cream without considering the underlying causes. Even if the treatment works for the rash, the primary condition still exists. But the rash is a warning sign and could indicate a serious problem in organs like the liver or digestive system. Covering the symptom only covers and perpetuates the problem. Even though all the symptoms we experience have a purpose, they have become demonized by our culture of symptomism.

We are called upon to wear pink ribbons and purple shirts so that we can all rally around the hope of finding a miracle cure that can fight off the evil disease. But most of the money raised and the subsequent research go toward more symptom suppressing medications — which could never resolve the original problem.

How else can we eradicate evil things like disease?

You can try to get rid of the flies with
fly catchers and poisons, or you can simply
clean up the garbage.
~ Dr. Reggie Gold

If the body is overstressed, toxic, or unhealthy, it becomes a wonderful breeding ground for any variety of diseases depending on one's genetic makeup. One option is to try and fight these lifestyle and environmentally related diseases — usually with medications. Another option is to restore the body to a healthy state. In fact, *it's a good idea to keep the body in a healthy state regardless of the onset of symptoms.*

Are You Listening?

In a wellness or holistic paradigm, symptoms are guideposts used to redirect our behaviors and create whatever change is needed in our lives.

These changes may need to come from the areas of:

- Nutrition
- Physical, chemical, or emotional stress
- Relationships
- Releasing old traumas
- Being in line with our purpose

Dr. Donald Epstein, one of my mentors, says, "The purpose of the symptom is to inspire change in behavior. The more intense the symptom, the more immediate and radical the internal transformation required."

The basic idea here is that our body is expressing symptoms to communicate to us that some sort of change in life is required. The wellness or holistic paradigm is all about recognizing symptoms as a call for change and exploring the messages they have for us.

The question then becomes: Why wouldn't we want to treat the symptom?

I am not suggesting that the symptoms never need to be treated; however, I do suggest that we look a little deeper into the message that a symptom may be trying to give us.

Perhaps we need:

- More sleep
- Less stress
- To eat better
- To experience more peace or joy

Maybe traumatic events in our lives have caused us to become disconnected from our bodies, and it's time to become whole again. Perhaps our soul has a purpose that we are not fulfilling, and the symptoms being expressed are its way of communicating that to us.

Symptomism

Today, many people use natural methods like chiropractic, acupuncture, or nutrition, and plug them into the failing system of symptom suppression. Even if these methods are *natural,* if the intent is only to treat symptoms, we're still working in a failed paradigm.

Contrary to popular opinion, our medical system is not failing because medical practitioners use harmful synthetic drugs or invasive surgical procedures—although they don't always help the situation. The system is failing because the focus is solely on silencing the symptoms. Ultimately, the body cannot be shut up forever and the symptoms will inevitably return—or another, more extreme symptom will be expressed to initiate change.

One thing's for sure; I'm not going to be the practitioner who attempts to shut off the warning signals. There are already plenty of practitioners doing that.

In our culture of symptomism, we also tend to suppress the symptoms of our lives. We often use alcohol, drugs, food, TV, and social media to escape from our stresses. Of course, just like in health, you can't cover the symptoms forever. Ultimately, regardless of our attempt to avoid them, all situations come to head. In life, it may be a deterioration and eventual end of a relationship. But when it comes to our health, our body continues to break down while we cover up the warning signs, leading to further deterioration of health, worsening of symptoms, and premature aging and death.

CHAPTER TWO

Why Is Health Declining?

STRESS

The Root of the Problem

If I had to pick one thing above all other things that leads to poor health, it would be stress. When people think of stress, they typically think of the boss driving them crazy with deadlines in combination with their family concerns. It would be more accurate to call these events *stressors*. Stressors typically consist of life events like work stress, divorce, and loss of a loved one, but can also include environmental and chemical factors as well.

Stress is the physiological response that the body has to stressors. Most of us are aware of what is happening in our body when we are under major stress. We can feel it — our muscles tighten, our breath becomes more shallow, and our heart rate increases.

Sometimes, stress is not so noticeable. We can become anesthetized to lower-level stressors or even major stressors that go on for long periods. As an old story goes, if you drop a frog into boiling water, it will immediately jump out. If you put a frog into room temperature water and slowly turn up the heat, it doesn't notice what is happening until it's too late. Many people are just like the boiling frog when it comes to stress.

During times when you are experiencing emotional or mental stress, you're either thinking of what happened in the past or what may or may not happen in the future. This can also be called *psychological stress*. It is a lot like reacting to a scary movie; your body's physiology doesn't know that it is not real.

Similarly, when you replay events from the past or imagine future scenarios in your mind, your body responds as if those imagined events are happening in the moment. Consider that most of the time, your mind is perpetually living in the future or the past. You are potentially in stress mode all the time.

Survival Mode

What is the problem with being in stress mode all the time?

I had the opportunity to visit Tuscany a few years back. Many of the cities, originally settled in ancient Roman times, were built with a wall around them to fight off enemies. Imagine that you lived in one of these cities during the time it was built, and you were about to be attacked. You and your fellow citizens may drop your normal activities — the blacksmith or farmer drop their tools — pick up weapons, and get on the wall to defend the city. Now imagine, even after the attack is over, the citizens stayed on the walls defending.

What if much of the city kept most of its resources tied up in defense for survival?

How productive would the city be?

When your mind is stuck in the past or the future, you are stuck in stress mode all the time, just like the example of the Tuscan city. Your energy and resources are tied up in stress physiology. It's perfectly normal for your body to respond this way to stress, but perpetual or long-term stress can lead to or exacerbate just about any health condition.

What's happening here?

First, some basic biology: You have a nervous system that is like a wiring system, sending and receiving signals to and from different parts of your body. Part of that nervous system is under voluntary control. This allows you to move the muscles in your legs and arms and engage in activities like chewing and swallowing.

The automatic nervous system is the part that is outside of our voluntary control. It controls our glands and organs, signaling them to release their hormones, which control all the body's functions. Imagine having to constantly monitor and control the functions of the stomach, liver, and heart. You would never get anything else done.

The automatic nervous system has two basic functional parts: the sympathetic nervous system and the parasympathetic nervous system. The parasympathetic nervous system directs the body to slow down, rest, digest, and heal while the sympathetic nervous system kicks in when it's time to get up and go.

When you perceive an event as stressful, the sympathetic nervous system kicks in, and the body goes into fight-or-flight mode. Stress hormones like cortisol are released, increasing the body's blood flow, heart rate, and energy so you can fight or run. The problem is that fight-or-flight physiology is only meant to be a short-term strategy.

Anyone who experiences chronic stress knows how it depletes energy and negatively affects digestion, sleep, our immune system, and just about everything else. Long-term stress can contribute to heart disease, diabetes, and even premature aging. It can also affect how our brain works.

I Can't Process This!

You may notice that when you're stressed, you're also less able to figure things out. This is because stress diminishes the cognitive functions of the brain. When you are stressed, you're not as creative as you could be, not as loving, and less able to relate to others. When you are already stressed, you will have a hard time adapting to future stresses and will have difficulty with adaptation in general.

I can remember several occasions of being stressed and frustrated while trying to figure out an accounting glitch. No matter how many times I went over the numbers, I couldn't figure out the solution. When I came back to it later, and I wasn't so stressed, it was amazing how easy it was to identify the problem and solve it.

Have you ever heard someone say: *I just can't deal with this right now?*

What they are really saying is that they don't have the available resources to process the amount or content of information.

Why?

Because when we are in fight-or-flight stress physiology, it is not the right time for love, creativity, or to think: *wow, that is a beautiful flower.* It's a time for survival—a strategy handled by the less-evolved brain.

If you were attacked, you wouldn't have time to use the frontal cortex to try to figure out the complexities of the situation. In times of stress, your resources are directed away from the frontal cortex, which explains the challenges in adapting to life changes when stressed.

When we evaluate an individual's case at our clinic, determining the underlying causes of the chronic health issue is part of the puzzle; making lifestyle changes and addressing the need to improve health is the other. In addition to evaluating the damage stress has on the function of the body, we recognize that it can also paralyze problem solving in people desperate to make healthier lifestyle choices. So, it is essential that chronic stress is addressed if one is to successfully improve their health.

POOR CHOICE

What We Eat

I used to take the New York State Thruway to and from college. Fast food was the only option available on the toll road. It wasn't long before I realized that every time I ate the food, I felt crappy. From that point on, I stopped eating at fast food joints.

That was about thirty years ago. Since that time, plenty of information has been made available about how bad fast food is for our health. Nevertheless, I never cease to be amazed at the line of cars waiting to get into the McDonald's. Health is a matter of choice.

We are what we repeatedly do.
Excellence, then, is not an act, but a habit.
~ Aristotle

Every day we make choices that either add to or detract from our health. It's not that any one choice is the make or break of anyone's health. Rather, it's the cumulative effect of our choices that shape our health. Sometimes, we make choices we know are unhealthy, and other times, we think we are making healthy choices when we are in fact making poor ones. For example, some clients are under the mistaken impression that egg yolks are bad because of the cholesterol, or that diet coke, margarine, and gluten-free alternatives are actually healthy choices.

When I ask most clients how they eat, they say they eat well. Then, I have them fill out a food journal. After a week or so, we'll go over it and see where we can improve. An overwhelming majority of the time, they say something like: *This is a bad week.*

After a few weeks of the same, they come to the realization they are not eating as well as they could or thought they were. Sometimes, it's things like candy and desserts that they know aren't good. Aside from that, there are usually several foods that they think are good but aren't.

In second grade, I remember learning about the food pyramid. The largest section was on the bottom and consisted of breads and grains. Judging from the food journals I look at, just about everyone else learned the same food pyramid. *That version of the food pyramid was completely wrong.* It has nevertheless had a huge impact on our collective eating habits and our overall health.

In the early 1900s, we began to see the introduction and steady increase of processed foods. While some processing in foods is not bad, we have gotten to the point where most of our foods are processed with chemical preservatives, trans fats, flavoring, and artificial sweeteners.

In 1939, Dr. Weston Price published, *Nutrition and Physical Degeneration*. Essentially, Dr. Price traveled to various isolated parts of the Earth where inhabitants had no contact with civilization and studied their health and physical development. Price found tribes or villages where virtually every individual exhibited genuine physical perfection. In other words, they did not have any chronic diseases common in western society.

Dr. Price also found that when people from these various cultures were influenced by the modern processed-food diet, they would also develop Westernized diseases. While the diets of these various cultures differ, they had in common the shared similarity of a diet of wholesome, nutrient-dense foods.

Over a ten-year period beginning in 1932, a medical doctor named Francis Pottenger conducted a series of revealing experiments with cats. Essentially, one group of cats was fed a natural diet while the other group was fed a processed-food diet. With each generation, the processed-food cats became more and more riddled with chronic disease, while the natural food cats thrived.

Dr. Pottenger said, "While no attempt will be made to correlate the changes in animals studied with malformations found in humans, the similarity is so obvious that parallel pictures will suggest themselves."

If we look at what has happened to the health of our society, we've become like the fourth generation of Pottenger's cats. As we face a generational decline of the health in this country, it's safe to say that Dr. Pottinger was on to something. We are eating plenty of food, but we are nutritionally starving.

A Slow Poisoning

No person in their right mind would choose to poison themselves. But that's what most of us do every day whether we are aware of it or not. Even smokers realize choosing to smoke comes with consequences for their health. People choose not to smoke because of the negative health consequences, yet they unknowingly choose to expose themselves to many other toxic substances.

When I was about four years old, I decided my mom's perfume smelled good, so good that

I thought it must taste good too. Boy, was I wrong. I also didn't realize at the time that the perfume was made of toxic chemicals, and they are certainly not good to drink.

What if we were to breathe in those chemicals through our lungs day after day?

It would get into our bloodstream the same as if we drank it or let it soak into the skin. Speaking of soaking into the skin, when the air gets cold and dry, the number of cases we see of chemical stress due to petroleum solvents always increases. Moisturizing creams, make-up, nail polish and remover, deodorants, and antiperspirants are filled with toxic chemicals. Yet, many people apply them daily without knowing that they are slowly poisoning themselves.

It's tough to get away from all these toxins we use without a second thought. Most people wash their clothes, and most of them are using detergents that are toxic and never really rinse completely out. Speaking of washing, most people use soap, shampoo, and even conditioner; of course, you wouldn't want to ingest them, but they do soak into the skin. Most have smells — those nasty perfume chemicals again.

Pharmaceutical companies are among the most profitable businesses in the world. That's because a lot of people are using their products. Sometimes, medications are necessary to control a symptom like keeping blood pressure from rising too high. The downside of medications is that they will never correct the underlying cause of a problem, and they are chemicals. Like most chemicals, they are toxic to the body. That's why all medications also have undesirable outcomes called side effects.

Often during a consultation, a patient will state that they hate taking medication. After talking a bit more, they will say something like: *Well, sometimes I take a little Tylenol, but only for headaches a couple times a week. And Tums for when I eat certain foods that upset my stomach. Sometimes, I take something if I need to get some sleep.* Because these over-the-counter drugs are so common, people often don't even realize that they're using medications.

You may think since the Food and Drug Administration (FDA) allows all these products, they are safe. It is true. You might not drop dead on the spot. It is a cumulative effect of all the chemicals over weeks, months, and years that causes deterioration of the body and loss of health.

Sedentary Society

It's no secret that our society has become sedentary. You may have heard that sitting is the new smoking. According to a study conducted by the Annals of Internal Medicine, more sedentary time means increased mortality. It can be challenging to avoid this pitfall. We spend a good portion of our childhood behind a desk and a good portion of our adulthood behind a computer.

And, what do we do after work?

For many, it's more time siting while on our Facebook pages or catching our favorite TV shows, and the list goes on. There are plenty of distractions to keep us sedentary.

What about the kids after they come home from school and sit down for an hour or two of homework?

For many of our children, it's a few more hours of video games or watching TV.

Although I have some ideas as to how and why being sedentary affects health and longevity, science isn't yet clear on exact mechanisms. One thing's for sure. It most definitely has a negative impact.

OUR ENVIRONMENT

It's a Dirty World

Pollution is defined by the American Heritage Science Dictionary as: "the contamination of air, water, or soil by substances that are harmful to living organisms."

In 2012, the World Health Organization estimated that one in eight global deaths is related to air pollution. While arguably a necessary evil of modern society, industry and its resulting pollution have added, and continue to add more and more toxins to the environment. Each year 1.2 trillion gallons of untreated sewage, stormwater, and industrial waste are dumped into U.S. waters.[1]

Every year, billions of pounds of toxic chemicals are dumped into the environment. In fact, in 1989, the Environmental Protection Agency (EPA) estimated that 5.7 billion pounds of chemicals were dumped in the public sewage or released into the ground, surface waters, or air. Imagine the cumulative effect of that much pollution over the decades.

In 2015, the EPA estimated that 40 percent of the lakes in America are too polluted for fishing, aquatic life, or swimming.[2] If these toxins are

1   Chambers, Neil B. "How Infrastructure Makes Water Work for Us." *Urban Green: Architecture for the Future.* Palgrave Macmillan, 2011. 37.
2   US Environmental Protection Agency. "Nonpoint Source Pollution: The Nation's Largest Water Quality Problem." Web accessed April 25, 2015.

in the water supply, they are everywhere else as well.

In modern times, it is literally impossible to shield yourself from the multitude of toxins in your environment. Even your organic garden is subject to the toxins that rain down from the sky.

It's not only the human-made toxins we have to contend with in the environment. For instance, the groundwater where I live has high levels of arsenic. Although arsenic is a naturally occurring heavy metal, it creates health problems nevertheless. Every area has its own set of potential toxins from naturally occurring sources.

As bad as it sounds outdoors, the environment inside our homes can be even worse. Gases from building materials, carpets, paint, fire retardants on furniture, HVAC systems, radon, and personal products we may use like candles or household cleaners can all contribute to poor air quality in the home.

A Heavy Toll

When it comes to discussion of why we are losing our health, I would be remiss if I didn't mention heavy metal toxins like mercury and aluminum. Mercury is by far the most common toxicity I find when evaluating a patient. Environmental mercury can come from fluorescent light bulbs, batteries, various industrial processes, and last but not least, silver fillings in teeth.

While most people now choose composite fillings for their teeth, the use of silver metal fillings began in the 1800s and continues today. At this point, generations of people have had silver fillings and the associated toxicity that goes along with it. After many years of testing clients for mercury toxicity, I have concluded that if you have, have had, or were born to a mother with silver fillings, you have mercury toxicity. It is beyond epidemic; it is pandemic.

Over the years, I have helped people with mercury detoxification, and often thought of renaming my clinic the Mercury Detox Center.

Mercury is a significant contributor to poor health in this society.

Aluminum is another example of an extremely common heavy metal toxicity we find. Consider the widespread use of aluminum-containing antiperspirants in our culture. Exposure can also come from cookware, food storage, and foil. Mercury and aluminum, along with numerous other metals, can cause immune suppression, tissue damage, and a general decline in health. Even metals like copper and zinc, which we require in trace amounts, can cause problems if optimal levels are exceeded.

FRANKENFOODS

Today, most patients I ask have at least heard of genetically modified organisms, or GMOs. Beyond that, they don't know much else because the issue is mostly swept under the rug. GMOs are created in a lab by cross-engineering a genetic line of a plant or animal in ways that normally wouldn't happen in nature.

One example of this is Monsanto's corn. The corn is genetically modified to be resistant to herbicides. Of course, the more herbicides can be used, the more herbicides are used, and that translates to a plant that is more toxic. It's interesting to note the crops subjected to the most genetic modification—corn, soy, and wheat—are the main ingredients for most of the packaged and processed foods that Americans love to eat.

Companies like Monsanto insist the GMOs are safe, but that's what they said about DDT and Agent Orange. The fact is, they can't be trusted to deliver unbiased information on the safety of their products. Also, because the government agencies like the FDA are influenced by government lobbyists from companies like Monsanto, we can't count on them to protect us either.

In our office, we test clients for food sensitivities. You can probably guess which are the most common foods that show up. That's right: wheat, soy, corn, and sugar. The American Academy of Environmental Medicine urges doctors to prescribe *non-GMO diets for all patients.* They cite animal studies showing organ damage, gastrointestinal immune disorders, accelerated aging, and infertility.

CHAPTER THREE

Health Impact

OUCH, THAT HURTS!

According to the 2003 edition of *The Physician's Desk Reference,* health is a state characterized by:

- Anatomical, physiological, and psychological integrity

- Ability to perform personally valued, family, work, and community roles

- Ability to deal with physical, biological, psychological, and social stress

- Feelings of well-being and freedom from the risk of disease and untimely death

Notice this definition goes way beyond the mere absence and presence of disease. It probes into how the loss of health is connected to our perceptions, our ability to adapt to stress, and our ability to contribute to our community. These are the things that really matter. It's not the diagnosis; it's how it affects your life.

Quite a Loss

When it comes to the loss of health, each person has a unique set of contributing ingredients, yet, the basic recipe is similar in most cases:

- Stress
- Toxicity
- Lack of adequate nutrition

As a child, I remember being healthy. Every year, I would get an award for having perfect attendance for the school year. I never thought that it could happen until one day in my mid-thirties, I realized I was losing my health. My body was stressed, toxic, and malnourished. Looking back, there were signals along the way, but I didn't pay attention to them.

When I began to lose my health, I carried between twenty and thirty extra pounds. I began to get colds and flus more frequently, and I didn't have as much energy. My feet would begin to hurt by simply walking on the hard floor of the grocery store. I didn't know it at the time, but I was experiencing the slow progression of my body breaking down. Cells that make up the tissues that make up the organs were toxic, malnourished, and dying.

For many, this early stage of health loss is experienced as *an annoyance that can easily be quelled by a medication,* at least for a while.

The Pain and the Drain

Even if we can contain or cover up the symptoms for a time, without resolution of the root cause, health will continue to deteriorate. Each person's chronic health condition is determined by which of their organs are breaking down. The eventual commonality of most chronic health conditions is pain.

Pain undoubtedly drives a lion's share of the billions of pharmaceutical sales in this country. Headaches, arthritis, neck and back pain, fibromyalgia, or any of the myriad of inflammatory and autoimmune diseases leave many people feeling like they have no choice but to reach for a pain reliever.

The effects of chronic pain go beyond physical discomfort. Sometimes, I was in too much pain to get out of bed. That wasn't so bad. It was the times when I could still get out of bed and work through the pain that were worse. Being in pain all day is draining. You could see the exhaustion on my face at the end of the day.

Of course, pain is not the only health issue that will sap your energy. Poor sleep, low blood sugar issues, a tired thyroid, and worn-out adrenals can all contribute to the energy drain that will leave you fully depleted by the end of the day, if not earlier. It's no wonder the loss or lack of energy is almost always one of the top two concerns listed on a patient's intake forms. When we barely have energy to get through the day, we generally don't have much left over for anything else — like the fun stuff.

When You Don't Feel Like Playing

It may sound strange, but most people don't really care what their diagnosis is. What really matters is how health affects one's participation in life.

There have been many occasions in my life when, because of ailing health, I was unable to do the things I wanted. When my knee was the size of a football, it made just about everything more difficult, if not impossible. So, I would bow out and make some excuse why I couldn't go to the outdoor concert or to play Frisbee. Slowly, as my health worsened, I went from an active lifestyle to being almost completely sedentary. Ice hockey, skiing, soccer, and even the ability to run across the yard began to slip away.

I got to the point where I began to miss weeks at a time from the office. Even when I could make it in, it wasn't pretty. As you can imagine, limping around the office was not a great practice builder. I began to think about what I could do from a wheelchair. I enjoyed writing and playing guitar. But then my wrists and fingers also began to fall victim to the painful joint swelling that was taking over every part of my life.

If we don't get to the root of the problem, our chronic health conditions don't usually get better. As they get worse, we participate less, and that can be depressing.

HOW DO YOU FEEL ABOUT THAT?

About two days before the intense pain and swelling stage, I could feel it. It was almost imperceptible, yet I knew it was coming.

As soon as I felt that subtle shift happening, my emotional state would shift to anxiety about what was soon to unfold:

- How long would it go on?
- How many days would I have to close the office?

- How painful was it going to be?
- What would my patients think?

In addition to the physical symptoms of inflammation, pain, and exhaustion, the repeating cycle of autoimmune flare-ups caused me a significant amount of emotional pain. I even felt shame because, despite my best efforts, I couldn't figure out how to get myself well.

Emotional Instability

When I opened my private practice in 1994, I was amazed at how many of my patients were on Prozac or some other mood-altering medication. What was interesting was that they didn't even think that this was a health problem. It had become such a norm in our society for people to suffer with mental illness.

Emotional instability, poor memory and focus, depression, and anxiety are more common than not. Emotional pain can be as bad or worse than physical pain for some. Emotional states like depression or anxiety can be the results of ailing health or how we feel about our poor health.

The brain, like the heart, pancreas, or liver, is an organ. Just like the rest of the organs, its functions — like focus, memory, and mood — are influenced by toxicities and nutrition. When we are experiencing depression or anxiety, it's not just a mental thing, it's a health problem.

It's tough to say that life situations don't influence how we feel, but someone with a healthy body and a healthy brain will handle the stresses of life better than someone whose brain is toxic and malnourished. Alcohol is an example of a toxin that can alter brain function. Just ask someone who has a bad hangover how their brain is functioning — or how it was functioning the night before.

Usually, when someone is experiencing emotional instability, it's a combination of factors. Chronic physical illness, like pain, can wear us down emotionally. That is especially true when the symptoms are unrelenting or progressing. We have all had the thoughts: *It feels like this is never going to end. No one can help me.* Essentially, we can lose hope. That is why we are willing to take medications to stop the pain.

I never really wanted to take medications, but the pain was competing with the things I needed to do, like work. So, I started with a little ibuprofen. After all, everybody does that. Of course, as time went on, the amount and frequency kept increasing. It helped some with the pain, but now I could add kidney and liver damage to my already extensive health issues.

Waning Motivation

Throughout the decade following my health decline, I looked for the answers to my health problems and experienced many emotional ups and downs. It would be more accurate to call them hopes and downs. I believed my body was capable of healing. I had many friends in the world of natural healthcare and numerous opportunities to pursue various healing modalities.

Yet, with each new hope came a new disappointment when I felt the next episode coming. Between the sporadic episodes of hope, I felt depressed about how my deteriorating health was affecting my quality of life. I was anxious about how I would be able to function and whether I would be able to continue my work. When my joints hurt, I felt old and inadequate, but most of all, I was embarrassed.

Sometimes, we can become disheartened when trying to reclaim our health. This is especially true when our efforts don't bring *immediate results*. Even though we might be on the right path, a lack of results can discourage us from continuing. And then it happens—we lose hope. This is perhaps the worst part because once we lose hope, we give up taking steps to improve our health, and we seal our fate. We slip into the world of symptom management and a lifetime of prescriptions.

Diminishing Confidence

I mentioned previously that lack of energy is one of the top two complaints patients list on their intake forms. The other is the desire to lose weight. Excess weight comes with a correlation to other health issues, like high blood pressure, diabetes, cancer, and heart disease. But that is not the main reason they are concerned. Their concern is how weight affects their appearance and how it makes them feel about themselves.

Weight loss is a twenty-billion-dollar industry, and women buy 85 percent of the products. They want to look better. Let's face it, we are a society that is obsessed with the way we look, and there is some merit to that. An individual's outside appearance—weight, skin, or even their vibrancy—are strong indicators of what is happening on the inside.

The bottom line is this—if we don't like our appearance, we are automatically more self-conscious and less confident. That can affect our relationships, our career success, and perhaps our happiness too.

BREAKING THE BANK

There is a cost to taking care of our health, just as there is a cost to not taking care of our health. Everyone is going to pay. Either we invest a small amount in our health now, or we pay a huge price along the way and in the end. That price includes more than just medical costs. It's not how long you live that matters most, but the quality of your life until you die.

> *If you think organic is expensive,*
> *have you priced cancer lately?*
> ~ Joel Salatin
> Founder, Polyface Farms

Healthcare Costs

Healthcare has been a hot news topic. While the health of this country spirals downward, healthcare costs continue to rise, and lawmakers scramble to figure out who is going to pay for it. Premiums and deductibles have nowhere to go but up. The symptom-management system that we refer to as healthcare is a house of cards that will eventually crumble and probably bankrupt the country on its way down.

You'd think that either losing a job, getting divorced, or being hit with an unexpected expense would be the top reason for going bankrupt. But do a search, and you'll see that medical expenses top them all. You'd probably also think that most of those cases were uninsured, but it is the opposite. Most are insured.

The idea that having insurance will protect your health and your finances is simply not true. I'd go as far as to say that having health insurance can make people less proactive about taking care of themselves and can even result in worse health.

Fiscal Fiasco

Insurance premiums and copays aren't the only ways we pay. Loss of health can negatively impact our financial outlook on several fronts. Those of us who are self-employed know that if we miss work, we don't get paid. Whether we work for ourselves or someone else, our health is intimately tied to our financial success.

Remember, chronic health conditions rob us of our energy, creativity, and productivity. As an employee, that can be the difference between who moves up and receives promotions in the company and who doesn't. For the self-employed, it can be the difference between being successful and being out of business.

On the days I was in a lot of pain, I would secretly hope in the back of my mind that that day wouldn't be too busy. Wouldn't you know it, that is exactly what would happen. Patients would cancel in droves. Between that and simply not having enough energy to sufficiently run the office, my finances suffered greatly.

It's All About Family

Perhaps the most egregious impact a loss of health can have is on our loved ones. If your health is affecting how you feel, your mood, energy level, or perhaps your sex drive, then you can bet it's also affecting your significant other, kids, friends, or coworkers. Loss of health can put strain on and even deteriorate a relationship.

It's typical for mothers to put everyone else's needs above their own, many times at the expense of their own health. The problem is that when they begin to lose their health, energy, and everything that goes along with it, they can't be their best self or contributor to their family. As they say, you can't give what you don't have.

Many people have experienced the stress of dealing with aging and sickly parents. It's hard to watch loved ones suffer. Brain disorders like dementia and Alzheimer's can be particularly challenging. It can also be taxing logistically and financially to take care of them. Personally, I'd like to do everything I can to maintain my best possible health and not put my kids through that.

Before I took the necessary steps to regain my health, I spent many a day unable to get out of bed. In addition to her already full plate, my wife Castine would prepare and serve all my meals and bring me anything else I needed. By the end of the day, she was worn out. By the end of the week, she was stressed out.

Castine would look at me and say, "You need to get better."

"I know, honey," I'd say.

CHAPTER FOUR

Steps to Regaining Health

AWARENESS

Much of the information in this chapter is also available by visiting my clinic's webpage, which is referenced at the end of the book.

While I'm pretty sure just about everyone wants to be healthy, the reality is that many people make daily choices to ensure poor health.

Why?

This is the critical question to ask if we have any chance of bettering our health personally and collectively.

Individuals who have reclaimed their health have some common attributes:

1. Awareness of what is happening in their body and why

2. Desire to do whatever is necessary to reach their health goals

3. A route or road map to reach their health goals

Collective Unconscious

Most of my time is spent coaching patients on healthy nutrition, lifestyle choices, and the impact that will have on present and future health. The first critical step for anyone desiring better health is to become *aware*. It's amazing, yet understandable, that many people aren't even aware they have health issues.

I was in denial about my own health for years. At first, the symptoms were tolerable. They got worse, but it wasn't all the time. Of course, as time went on, the frequency increased, and slowly it became more the norm than not. Somewhere along the line, I realized the pain and arthritis weren't going to magically disappear.

Chronic health issues can develop so gradually as to escape our notice. This is compounded by the cultural obsession with taking and doing things to numb ourselves from the reality of what is really happening to our health or life. Just turn on the TV, and in a short while, you will be bombarded with the advertising of pharmaceutical solutions for anything you could possibly feel, physically or mentally.

We have been programmed to cover over symptoms of declining health and any investigation of cause. This is a key component to the culture of symptomism. Overcoming the systematic numbing of awareness to an existing problem is the first step toward creating health.

What's Our Focus?

After realizing that there is a problem, we must change our focus from symptom suppression to investigating the underlying causes. Simply put, if we don't know what caused a problem, it's unlikely that we can resolve it.

In our office, we offer a curriculum that delivers information about proper nutrition, finding sources of health-destroying toxins, and how to effectively thrive in the presence of stress. Many chronic health problems can be traced back to one or more root causes that has overstressed the body, keeping it from being able to experience its full and glowing health.

Ingesting, breathing in, and soaking in toxic poisons could certainly cause enough stress to have a negative effect on the proper function of a human being. Insufficiency of one's dietary nutrition could cause great stress as well. The body's need for nutrients is indisputable.

Mental and emotional stress can be both a causative and exacerbating factor in all disease processes. We find that in most cases, it's all the above-mentioned factors that are impacting our clients' health.

Thanks to modern technology, most of the information about potential underlying causes is available on the internet. The potential pitfall here is that different sources can and frequently do give conflicting information. It's great to have all this health information available at our fingertips, but that doesn't mean it's accurate. I've seen this lead to uncertainty and inaction in individuals trying to regain their health. You would think that with everything we know, the overall health of our society would naturally improve. Not so.

What's missing?

Wisdom

While having information is great, figuring out what to do with that information — and then acting on it — is vital to regaining and maintaining health. Without putting knowledge into action, it is essentially useless. Taking actions that best serve your health requires you to examine the available information and discern which ideas to use and which to discard.

Throughout our lives, we are constantly gathering information. Some is gathered through first-hand experience, and some is what I would call intellectual information.

This type of information is incorporated into our belief system after we read about it or learn about it from another person. While intellectual information can be an extremely valuable, it can be a hindrance at times, especially if the information we're getting is incomplete or false.

Reading about something on the internet or hearing about it on a TV commercial doesn't necessarily make it true. We must consider the source of the information when determining its validity.

For instance, many of us who grew up watching cartoons on Saturday morning will remember the breakfast cereal commercials. According to the commercials, the cereals, fortified with eight essential vitamins and minerals, were a healthy part of a complete breakfast. The reality is that no breakfast cereal full of sugar, processed carbohydrates, preservatives, and food dyes is a healthy part of anything—even and especially if it's fortified with synthetic vitamins.

With all this conflicting and ever-changing information, how do we know what to believe and what to do?

Wisdom does not mean having all the answers; it means using critical thinking skills to ask the right questions:

- Does it make sense?
- Who is conducting the study?
- What do they have to gain?
- What are the long-term effects?

Wisdom can be gained by experience or shared from others who have had experience. By benefitting from others' experiences, our timeline to figure things out can move much faster. I spent years trying to figure out my health before getting help from people who had already walked the path. Sometimes, it takes having a little faith in a trusted source.

True wisdom can only be gained through your life experience. Once you have experienced something, your mind moves from the realm of belief to one of knowing. If you can learn how to apply a common-sense viewpoint, listen to your body, trust your inner wisdom, and be guided by these forces, you will not be at the mercy of your beliefs or someone else's.

With heightened awareness, you can move onto the next critical step in achieving a healthy lifestyle.

DESIRE

Once we have realized that our health is diminishing, and we understand why, the next critical step is to act. I find that this is where many people encounter a great deal of difficulty. Even if they know what to do, they either can't get started, or they can't sustain their new healthy behaviors.

Overcoming Addictions

Often, we become so addicted to our unhealthy life choices that they work against us when we are attempting to make healthy lifestyle changes. Most Americans eat poorly. This creates a cultural addiction to continue the behavior, even if we know it's not good for us. Just ask a parent who is trying to keep sugar out of their child's diet at the next birthday party. The first obstacle, cultural addiction, can be extremely difficult to overcome. The next problem we have is the physiological addiction to unhealthy foods.

A patient once asked me, "Why do they put so much sugar in our foods?"

I can assure you it's no mistake. The producers of these foods know that sugar is addictive, and they want you addicted to their product. Studies suggest that sugar is more addictive than heroin and cocaine.

The next major addiction to overcome is the addiction to our own habits. Change of any kind seems to be one of the most difficult endeavors for us humans. Repeated habitual thoughts and actions become hardwired in the brain. The constant bombardment of advertisements asserts its influence beginning at early childhood and continues throughout our lives.

What does this all mean?

Even if we overcome these addictions, healthy lifestyle changes don't just happen without motivation. One must aspire to change the pendulum and create health.

Finding Motivation

When I work with a new patient, the first thing I want to know is what's important to them. Unless we can tap into their source of motivation, converting unhealthy habits to a healthy lifestyle is unlikely. After interviewing thousands of patients, I see that while individual motivations vary, there are some common themes.

The top five reasons to live a healthy lifestyle are:

1. *Inability to participate fully in life*: There are many occasions in my life when because of my ailing health, I was unable to do the things I wanted. Severe joint pain and swelling makes just about everything more difficult if not impossible. The

desire to do things that are fulfilling can be a powerful motivator to achieving a healthy lifestyle.

2. *Becoming a burden on family*: Many of my clients must deal with their own aging and sickly parents. While they do so with compassion and a loving heart, they don't want their own children to deal with the same stresses, financial or otherwise, like they have with their parents.

3. *Cost of not taking care of health*: Everyone is going to pay. Either you invest a small amount in your health now or will pay a huge price in the end. That price includes more than just medical costs. It's not how long you live, but the quality of your life until you die.

4. *Feeling better*: Some people are just tired of feeling crappy. They are tired of taking medications that have worse side effects than the original problem. They have come to the realization that while it may temporarily reduce their pain, covering

their symptoms with drugs prevents them from achieving full and glowing health.

5. *Looking better*: This is one of the most popular reasons people seek a healthier lifestyle. Let's face it, we are a society obsessed with the way we look, and there is some merit to that. An individual's outside appearance — weight, skin, even vibrancy — are strong indicators of what is happening on the inside.

It's a Commitment

I remember on several occasions pleading with God to get me through the painful episodes of joint swelling. I promised that if He got me through, I'd quit eating sugar. Eventually, I got tired of repeating the pain cycle, and that became my motivation for making the change I so desperately needed.

Ultimately, motivation leads to commitment. The most accurate predictor of a patient's results is their level of commitment to getting well. When a patient thinks and says: *I'll do whatever is necessary to get well,* I know they are headed toward better health. All we need to do is point them in the right direction.

THE ROAD MAP

Imagine trying to get someplace that you have never been before without a GPS, road map, or even a compass. It would be a pretty daunting task. People who are successful in achieving a healthy lifestyle have a road map or route to get there.

Some people, by trial and error, figure out the steps necessary for them to create a healthy lifestyle. Some may require or desire a bit of guidance from those who have already figured it out. Most people fall somewhere in between. Without any kind of game plan, we all are almost sure to fail.

Three Steps to a Healthy Lifestyle

In determining our route to a healthier lifestyle, we want to remember to use the information gathering and critical thinking discussed earlier. Once we determine our goals, we can begin to take action by implementing three steps to creating our healthy lifestyle game plan.

1. *Set attainable goals*: The changes that we make must be realistic for us based on our lifestyles. If we set goals that are too difficult or even impossible to attain, then we increase the chance for failure. I found that for most people, small incremental changes are more sustainable than big life changes.

2. *Create some form of accountability*: This is where most people can use some help. Whether we do it on our own or with help, we need to have some system of keeping track of our goals to determine success. If needed, we can go back and make modifications to our plan.

3. *Realize there will be ups and downs*: As with any sustainable change, understanding this ahead of time can help keep us from going completely off the rails when we slip up. When this happens, it usually means our change was too abrupt, and we need to reexamine step one. I have never seen a progress graph of any kind that didn't have a few dips. Remember to keep the big picture in mind.

Executing the Plan

Sometimes, even if we have a well-thought-out plan for creating our healthy lifestyle, we still fail. There is one seemingly elusive step in achieving a healthy lifestyle — execution of the plan. When I witness a client struggling with this, it usually means they need assistance in directing their focus. Dr. Donald Epstein said, "all we can ever do is *determine where we place our focus.*"

Finding a method that caters to our strengths can help ensure our success in creating desired changes. Some people can create successful changes by participating in programs that focus on structure. Structures would include calendars, schedules, or steps. Twelve-step programs are an example of structure-based systems.

Other people do best when they focus their attention on perceptions first. Examples might include daily affirmations, visualizations, and motivational reassuring designed to alter feelings about themselves or their desired change.

Finally, there are some people who do best when they just get right down to doing it. They are better off not getting caught up in structures and perceptions.

Accessing Your Energy

If you find you have been previously unsuccessful with execution of lifestyle change, it does not mean that you are simply destined to fail. It more likely means that you haven't found the formula that best fits your individual style. You might even be sabotaging your process without knowing it. Don't worry, there is a key to achieving your goals.

Most of us have had the experience of doing well at something. If you ever achieved a goal with ease, you may have noticed that you had a higher level of energy. Subsequently, when we fail, our energy levels seem to be very low.

Which came first?

One of the most basic principles in physics states that change requires energy. Therefore, raising our level of energy can assist us in achieving the changes that we desire. Great!

Now, how do we do that?

Dr. Donald Epstein came up with a great road map to finding your own personal style of creating change. He calls it *reorganizational healing*. A triad linking perception, behavior, and structure makes up the foundation of this system. Understanding and optimizing the relationship that each side plays in our personal ability to make or adapt to changes can raise our energy level. It is in this state of heightened energy our goals can be met with much less effort.

Wouldn't that be nice?

If you haven't figured out how to make or stick to healthy lifestyle changes that you desire, don't give up. This is where most people need help and where having a mentor to guide them through the process is key. Consider that almost all successful people, from athletes to business executives, have a coach or mentor guiding them.

When it comes to our most precious asset — our health — doesn't it make sense to have some help?

CHAPTER FIVE

The Ripple Effect

PERSONAL BENEFITS OF HEALTH AND WELLNESS

What if instead of making choices only out of fear and avoidance of disease, we began to make transitions based on the possibility of our experience?

What if the decisions we make could enhance our life experience instead of only serving as a means of survival?

We can, but to accomplish this we must move out of the mainstream idea of health and into the realm of wellness. All the important things in life, including our relationships, our ability to enjoy our hobbies, create abundance, and experience a peaceful life are influenced and even dependent on our health.

Participating More Fully in Life

Handling stress, toxicity, nutrition, and moving toward better health will mean less overall inflammation. That means *less pain*. Let's face it, if you feel better, you're more likely to participate in all life has to offer. When your body feels good, you are much more likely to play, hike, and exercise. Life is a lot more fun when you can do what you want and participate fully.

Having the ability to actively move your body has some great side benefits as well:

- Activity helps to *keep* you healthy.

- Increased muscle strength and tone burns fat and strengthens bones.

- Increasing blood flow helps detoxify and brings oxygen to the body more effectively.

- Exercise and enjoyment increase chemical endorphins that help you achieve a higher state of mental and emotional health.

Thriving in Relationships

It's hard to be in a good mood when you're not feeling well or are in pain all the time. That discomfort is what motivates most of us to suppress the symptoms in the first place. When you begin to regain your health, the benefits go far beyond physical comfort.

Imagine walking around all day with a pebble in your shoe. By the end of the day, you're probably not the most pleasant person to be around. Getting healthy is like removing the pebble from your shoe, and that has a huge effect on how you relate to others. It's so much easier to connect and enjoy the company of others when we're not distracted by our pain.

Stress, toxicity, and lack of proper nutrition all have a negative effect on brain function. Improving health by handling these stressors reduces inflammation, which in turn has a positive impact on all cognitive functions of the brain. When our brain is healthy, we experience less depression and anxiety; we think more clearly; and our overall outlook becomes more positive. That's good for us, but it's also good for the people around us.

Several years ago, I gave up eating processed sugar to help reduce the amount of pain I was in. It worked, but there was also a side benefit that I wasn't aware of previously. Before removing sugar, I experienced what I thought were normal ups and downs. Some days my mental state was good, and other days, I felt down for no particular reason. It wasn't until a few months passed without any more down days that I realized the impact sugar had. Many years later, and still, no more down days.

When we're feeling better and have a positive outlook, our relationships improve. We're no longer dragged down by the drama and addictions that go hand in hand with poor brain health, which leaves us more energy to direct toward those around us. It gives us the opportunity to thrive in our relationships.

Creating an Abundant Life

In life, whatever we focus our attention on tends to expand. If we focus on all the bad things in life, we end up with a crappy life. If we focus on the good, we tend to attract more of the same. We can literally create our reality by how we think. The brain is a powerful tool, but like the rest of the organs, is subject to toxicities, malnutrition, and inflammation. When our body and brain are healthy, it's much easier to stay positive and focus our attention in a way that serves us.

It's no coincidence that people who are healthy tend to create the life that they want. They move out of the survival mindset and into one of abundance. When we realize we can take control of our own health, it's not much of a stretch to realize we can do the same with our life. The two, in fact, go hand in hand.

Chronic health issues sap our energy, leaving us with barely enough to make it through the day. When we improve our health, we tend to have much more energy available not only to get through the day, but to focus on improving other areas of our lives. Maybe we partake in some training or education so that we can get a better paying job. Maybe we start our own business, or learn how to invest, or even read a book that will help improve the quality of our lives. Whatever we decide to do, we are actively creating a more abundant life.

BEYOND THE PHYSICAL

Health and wellness transcend mere blood chemistry levels and the presence or resolution of physical symptoms. Wellness could be brought up as a continuum that offers ever-expanding benefits as we continue down its path.

The Wellness Continuum

Sometimes, we tend to think of health in black and white. Either we are sick, or we are not. But there are varying degrees of both health and wellness in either direction. Our health tends to describe the physical, biochemical function of the body; wellness, on the other hand, is more indicative of our mental and emotional perception about our health and life. On the illness end of the spectrum, we experience fear, distrust, helplessness, and isolation. On the wellness end of the spectrum, we experience love, trust, resourcefulness, and community.

Based on blood tests and lab values, you may get a clean bill of health but still feel like something is wrong or not working in your life. This is an example of supposedly good health but a lack of wellness.

What if someone received a major diagnosis like cancer?

They may react by shutting down and going into fear and isolation. That is an illness response. Or, they could say to themselves: *I am going to live and love and do everything I can in the time I have left*. That is an example of a wellness response, even in the presence of physical disease.

While our biochemical and physical experience of health is different from the emotional experience of wellness, they are inextricably connected. Wellness is naturally enhanced by building physical health beyond mere symptom management and ensuring proper lab values.

Adaptability

One major aspect of wellness is the ability to change and adapt. Adaptation is the key to life. In nature, if a species doesn't adapt, it ceases to exist. Businesses and corporations must constantly change and stay ahead of the curve to stay profitable. We as individuals must also adapt and change if we want to thrive in our lives.

As employees, those who can acclimate to changing business environments tend to perform better, ensure value in their position, and move up in the company. The difference between successful small businesses and those that fail is in their ability to change when something isn't working. Those who thrive in their relationships realize they must grow and adapt or their relationship will wither and die.

As discussed earlier, the stress physiology and inflammation that accompany ailing health limit our access to the frontal cortex. This more advanced part of our brain is responsible for love, creativity, and the ability to assess our situation and make appropriate changes. The lower brain centers are great for the repetitive actions in life, like brushing our teeth and even driving the car on a familiar route. But adapting to the ever-changing situations of life requires access to a well-functioning and available frontal cortex. As we improve our health and wellness, we naturally and spontaneously improve our ability to make the changes that will ultimately enhance our life experience.

Something I've realized through the experience of my own health journey is that it never ends. I am constantly learning new things and changing and adapting to continue to move toward greater levels of my own health and wellness. People who are well wouldn't have it any other way.

Making a Contribution

As we move toward the wellness end of the spectrum, we realize that it's not just about us. On the illness end of the spectrum, our focus is much narrower. Our tendency is toward reducing symptoms, trying to cope with stress, and just trying to make it through the day.

As we become healthier and increase our wellness, our focus opens beyond our own survival and moves naturally toward contribution. Most people I ask believe that they have a purpose in life. Most of the time, that purpose involves making a contribution to others or to the greater good. Those who don't or who haven't figured it out tend to feel lost. This is especially true when life's challenges come along. Contribution is a true litmus test of wellness.

However, contributing to others is difficult, if not impossible, if we don't first take care of ourselves. We must have the energy, resources, and fruits of our own abundance if we want to share it with others. Oftentimes, a mother will give everything she has to take care of her family while neglecting her own health, not realizing in the long run that neglecting herself diminishes what she can contribute to her loved ones.

The consequences of being good custodians of our own health go far beyond personal benefit. I would argue that it is our responsibility to improve our health and wellness because then we can fully contribute our gifts to a world that desperately needs help.

THE RIPPLE EFFECT

As we experience greater levels of wellness, we begin to realize that every choice we make influences the entire web of life. Once we realize this, we begin to make more conscious choices, not only for our own personal health, but for the environment and others who share it. We realize that it's not just about us.

Our Environment

We'd have to be living under a rock not to realize how modern life has impacted the pollution in our environment. Complaining or hoping that our politicians will fix this problem won't work because it is the result of the collective choices we make every day.

Greater awareness is one of the attributes of wellness. As we move up the wellness continuum, we automatically make healthier choices for ourselves. But we must also realize that the choices we make have a positive or negative effect on the environment. Toxic chemical products we use every day can harm our health. But they also build up in the environment over time and end up in our food and water supply to come back around and continue to harm us and other species.

One of the most profound positive effects we can have on the environment is through our purchasing power. Complaining about large corporations that treat the environment poorly while we have filled their pockets by continuing to patronize their business is fruitless. We must consciously choose where we spend our money and what it will support.

When we make healthier choices for ourselves and for our families, we are supporting natural and organic businesses that are less harmful to the environment. At the same time, we are taking money from less environmentally-conscious companies, ultimately forcing them to change or go out of business.

The Food Supply

The large bulk of the American diet consists of highly-processed and packaged food products that are filled with added sugars, preservatives, flavor enhancers, food dyes, and sodium. Healthy people and those who are striving to be healthy realize they must cut out the processed and packaged foods and replace those with real, wholesome food.

Once again, our food buying choices also have *far-reaching effects*. Consuming organically grown products benefits our health by limiting the harmful fungicides and pesticides we take in. And, it also sends growers the message that the public wants cleaner produce. That message forces the market to adjust to the buying power of consumers.

Several years ago, I recall bringing a tomato home from the grocery store. I cut into it expecting the delicious taste of the juicy tomatoes we used to grow in our garden when I was a kid. What I got was something having a closer resemblance to cardboard.

What was missing?

Mainstream farming methods have stripped essential nutrients from the soil through overuse and improper crop rotation. Buying produce from local sources helps support our individual health, while at the same time contributing to more sustainable farming. By buying from local farms, we can get fresher foods from a known source while cutting out the environmental toll of transporting foods across the country.

For Generations to Come

Obviously, choosing a healthier lifestyle has a positive impact on your life. In addition to your loved ones, your choices have an impact on many people you haven't even met and will impact the lives of future generations as well.

Each year, more and more chemicals enter the environment, many of which can take decades to break down and dissipate. These chemicals can be found in the most pristine areas of the world.

The introduction of genetically modified organisms, or GMOs, has coincided with a general increase of health problems in this country. The most heavily modified crops just so happen to be the ones found in most packaged foods. While the companies that produce them assure their safety, no long-term independent studies exist to support those claims. In fact, many other countries have already banned their use.

Once these Frankenfoods have entered the environment, their seeds mix with other crops.

Once that happens, we can never go back. By using these foods, we could be inadvertently changing the genetics of our food supply forever.

Conclusion

The choices that we've made up until this point have determined where we are in our health and in our lives. The choices that we make from this point going forward will determine the outcome of our next five, ten, or fifteen years and beyond. But our choices go far beyond our own personal outcomes.

My father once said to me, "Either you're with God, or you're against Him."

My interpretation of my father's words is that we are all part of the web of life. Everything we do, every choice we make, contributes or detracts from life. Life is a gift, not to be squandered. The choices we make matter, not only to us and our own quality of life, but to those around us and the greater good as well. As we realize this, we understand that living a healthy lifestyle is a gift and a responsibility.

What do we do now?

At this point, I hope you've been inspired to improve your health and your life. I would encourage you to pull back the veil from the cultural story that tells us that medications are a normal and necessary part of our healthcare, getting older naturally means getting sicker, and that we should just settle for failing health as the norm. If we want different results than mainstream America, we must question the mainstream narrative.

We must:

- Research
- Gain multiple perspectives
- Learn to think critically
- Ask: *Is this logical? Does this make sense?*

Finally, we all must seek help. It's okay, and even essential, to ask for help from others who have experience in gaining, maintaining, and enhancing health and wellness. Seeking guidance will put you on the proper path, keep you motivated, and save you valuable time.

Remember, *improving health is a journey.* If we try to swallow it all in one bite, it can be overwhelming. Take it one step at a time. Maybe it's a small change in your diet, or ten minutes of stress reduction practice. There will be times where you feel like you are going backwards. Keep on the path, and you'll be sure to reap the rewards.

Next Steps

For more information on Dr. Clerkin, visit drgeneclerkin.com

call 603-852-4706, or

email dr.gene@monadnocknaturalhealth.com.

Be sure to like us on Facebook at Facebook.com/monadnocknaturalhealth.

About the Author

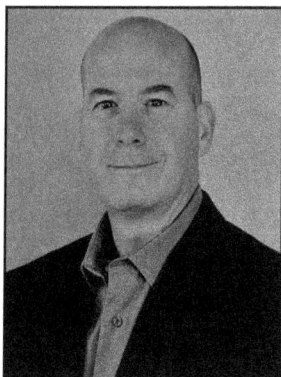

Dr. Gene Clerkin graduated from Life Chiropractic School in 1994 and opened his private practice soon after. Within a couple of years, he began to experience progressively worsening joint pain associated with an autoimmune condition. Dr. Clerkin got to the point where he could barely make it through the day. Finally, after more than a decade of intense pain and suffering, Dr. Clerkin learned how to uncover the root causes of his health problems and turn his health around using natural and effective solutions.

Feeling compelled to share his successful strategy with the many who suffer from metabolic disorders and chronic diseases, Dr. Clerkin went on to complete an advanced clinical training program in Nutrition Response Testing. In addition to adding clinical nutrition services to his chiropractic practice, he also realized that educating patients about supportive lifestyle changes was essential for them to be able to gain their health independence. Dr. Clerkin then added a healthy lifestyle curriculum as a cornerstone to his array of services.

Dr. Clerkin has also trained professionally with world-renowned human potential innovator, Dr. Donald Epstein, for over twenty years. By weaving what he has learned in clinical nutrition, chiropractic, and the field of healing, wellness, and human potential, Dr. Clerkin delivers a renowned humanistic approach to his wellness programs and his clients.